COMPLETE GUIDE TO UNDERSTANDING ROTATOR CUFF REPAIR

Comprehensive Insights On Diagnosis, Surgical Techniques, Rehabilitation, And Post-Operative Care For Shoulder Injuries

KLEIN HOYLE

Disclaimer

The content in this book is based on the author's expertise and comprehension of the topic. The author has no affiliation or link with any corporation, business, or person. This book is meant to give general information and educational material only, and it should not be interpreted as professional medical advice. Always seek the advice of a skilled healthcare expert if you have any queries about medical issues or treatments. The author and publisher expressly disclaim any responsibility resulting directly or indirectly from the use or use of the information included in this book.

Table of Contents

ABOUT THIS BOOK

The "Complete Guide to Understanding Rotator Cuff Repair" is an essential reference for anybody navigating the complexity of rotator cuff health and repair. This book begins with an in-depth look at the architecture of the rotator cuff and then goes on to explain the crucial functions and typical problems connected with this important shoulder component. Maintaining rotator cuff health is critical since it plays a role in total shoulder function and mobility.

Identifying rotator cuff injuries may be difficult, but this guide makes the process easier by outlining the signs to look for and the diagnostic procedures that are widely used, such as imaging methods. It also provides clear instructions on how to distinguish rotator cuff problems from other shoulder ailments and when medical intervention is required.

For individuals considering non-surgical treatment alternatives, this book covers a wide range of treatments, including physical therapy exercises to strengthen the shoulder, anti-inflammatory drugs, and corticosteroid injections. It also covers lifestyle and exercise changes that may help control symptoms and improve shoulder function without surgery.

Preparing for rotator cuff surgery entails several critical tasks, which this article painstakingly details. It provides a fair assessment of the risks and advantages of surgery, assisting patients in setting reasonable expectations for their recovery.

When surgery becomes essential, knowing the various surgical approaches is critical. This article discusses arthroscopic surgery, open surgery, and mini-open repair, as well as tips on how to choose the best strategy for each unique situation. Post-surgery recovery and rehabilitation are equally important, and this book gives a thorough plan for immediate post-operative care, physical therapy exercises, and pain management measures, all to assure a smooth recovery and prevent problems.

The various consequences and dangers of rotator cuff surgery are extensively explored, assisting patients in recognizing indicators of infection or re-injury, managing post-surgical stiffness, and understanding long-term results and prognosis. Another significant emphasis is on improving recovery and healing, including guidance on dietary assistance, the use of supplements and drugs, and the value of sleep and relaxation. The psychological components of healing are also addressed, recognizing the mental and emotional difficulties that patients may confront.

Returning to everyday activities and sports following surgery is a huge achievement, and this book offers practical advice for a gradual return to work and physical activity. Strategies for preventing re-injury and maintaining shoulder health, in the long run, are stressed, allowing patients to continue their busy lives without interruption.

Finally, long-term maintenance and prevention are essential for maintaining good shoulder health. This book provides regular shoulder strength workout regimens, flexibility maintenance strategies, and injury prevention advice. Regular check-ups and monitoring are essential to guarantee long-term shoulder health and early diagnosis of any problems.

CHAPTER 1

Introduction To The Rotator Cuff

Anatomy Of Rotator Cuff

The rotator cuff consists of four muscles and their tendons that surround the shoulder joint. These muscles and tendons act together to support the shoulder and allow for a variety of arm motions. The four muscles that form the rotator cuff are:

1. Supraspinatus: The supraspinatus muscle, located at the top of the shoulder blade, helps elevate the arm and stabilizes the shoulder joint.

2. Infraspinatus: The infraspinatus muscle, located underneath the supraspinatus, helps rotate the arm away from the body.

3. Teres Minor: This little muscle is underneath the infraspinatus and cooperates with it to rotate the arm externally.

4. The subscapularis muscle, located on the front of the shoulder blade, helps rotate the arm inward.

Each of these muscles is connected to the upper arm bone (humerus) by tendons, which create the rotator cuff. Tendons are prone to injury because they travel through a tight gap between the shoulder blade (scapula) and the humerus.

Functions Of Rotator Cuff

The main functions of the rotator cuff are:

1. The rotator cuff muscles and tendons stabilize the shoulder joint by firmly keeping the head of the humerus inside the scapula's shallow socket (the glenoid). This stability is essential for all shoulder motions and helps to avoid dislocations.

2. Rotator cuff muscles assist a variety of arm motions. The supraspinatus helps to elevate the arm to the side (abduction), while the infraspinatus and teres

minor are engaged in external rotation. The subscapularis aids in the internal rotation of the arm.

3. The rotator cuff tendons convey muscular force to the bones, allowing the arm to move with power and precision.

Understanding these roles emphasizes the need to maintain rotator cuff health for shoulder stability and mobility.

Common Injuries And Conditions

Several injuries and illnesses may damage the rotator cuff and impair its function. The most frequent are:

1. Tendinitis is inflammation of the rotator cuff tendons, which is often caused by overuse or repeated shoulder motions. This illness may cause discomfort and limited movement.

2. Bursitis is inflammation of the bursa, a fluid-filled sac that cushions the rotator cuff tendons. Bursitis is

often caused by excessive friction or pressure on the bursa.

3. Rotator Cuff Tear: Acute traumas, such as falls, or chronic deterioration may cause partial or full rips in the rotator cuff tendons. Tears may cause severe discomfort, weakness, and a loss of shoulder function.

4. Impingement Syndrome develops when the rotator cuff tendons get pinched or squeezed during shoulder motions, causing discomfort and irritation.

5. Calcific Tendinitis is the deposition of calcium deposits inside the rotator cuff tendons, which causes discomfort and inflammation. This syndrome may develop gradually or unexpectedly.

Importance Of Rotator Cuff Health

Maintaining the health of the rotator cuff is important for various reasons.

1. Preventing Pain: Strong rotator cuff muscles and tendons lower the likelihood of painful disorders like tendinitis and bursitis. Preventative interventions, such as adequate exercise and ergonomics, may help these tissues operate properly.

2. Ensuring Mobility: A robust and effective rotator cuff allows for a wide range of shoulder motions, which are required for everyday activities and physical demands. Without a strong rotator cuff, even basic tasks like reaching above or lifting items may become difficult.

3. Enhancing Athletic Performance: Athletes, particularly those who participate in activities that require repeated shoulder motions (such as baseball, tennis, and swimming), depend on a strong rotator cuff for peak performance. Rotator cuff strength, endurance, and resilience may all be improved with proper conditioning and training.

4. Strengthening and training the rotator cuff may reduce the chance of injury. Understanding and correcting risk factors, such as poor lifting methods or repeated strain, may help avoid rotator cuff injuries and impingement syndrome.

5. Facilitating Rehabilitation: For people recuperating from rotator cuff injuries, prioritizing rotator cuff health via physical therapy and tailored exercises is critical for restoring strength, flexibility, and function.

Individuals may preserve and strengthen the rotator cuff by studying its architecture, functions, frequent injuries, and the necessity of maintaining it.

CHAPTER 2

Recognizing Rotator Cuff Injuries

Symptoms Of Rotator Cuff Injuries

Rotator cuff injuries often cause several symptoms, which vary in intensity depending on the degree of the damage. The symptoms that are most common include:

• Common symptoms include shoulder discomfort and weakness that may spread down the arm. This ache usually worsens at night and might interfere with sleep. Weakness in the shoulder or arm is also prevalent, making it difficult to lift things or carry out daily chores.

• Reduced Range of mobility: Some individuals may have limited shoulder mobility. This might make it difficult to lift the arm, reach behind the back, or execute overhead tasks.

• Clicking or popping sensations when rotating the shoulder may suggest rotator cuff injury or impingement.

• Swelling and tenderness in the shoulder region may indicate inflammation or damage.

Diagnostic Tests And Imaging

Rotator cuff injuries must be diagnosed accurately to get effective treatment. Healthcare practitioners utilize a mix of physical tests and imaging tools to identify these ailments.

• Physical Exam: A doctor will evaluate the shoulder's range of motion, strength, and stability. They may use particular procedures, such as the Neer impingement test, Hawkins-Kennedy test, or drop arm test, to determine the site and severity of the injury.

• X-rays may detect bone spurs or other abnormalities that may contribute to the injury but do not show soft tissues such as rotator cuff tendons.

• The gold standard for diagnosing rotator cuff problems is Magnetic Resonance Imaging (MRI), which offers comprehensive pictures of soft tissues including muscles and tendons. It may reveal tears, inflammation, and other rotator cuff issues.

• An ultrasound may examine the rotator cuff by providing real-time pictures of the shoulder's soft tissues. It is a cheaper and more accessible alternative to MRI.

• Arteriogram: Injecting contrast dye into the shoulder joint before an X-ray or MRI may offer sharper pictures of the rotator cuff and possible tears.

Differentiating Rotator Cuff Injuries From Other Shoulder Issues

Rotator cuff injuries do not cause every case of shoulder discomfort. Distinguishing these injuries from other shoulder issues is critical for good therapy.

• Adhesive Capsulitis (Frozen Shoulder) produces discomfort and stiffness in the shoulder, comparable to a rotator cuff injury. However, a frozen shoulder usually causes a progressive loss of mobility in all directions, not only in particular actions.

• Shoulder impingement occurs when the shoulder blade scrapes on the rotator cuff tendons, producing discomfort and inflammation. While the symptoms coincide, shoulder impingement does not always result in a rotator cuff injury.

• Arthritis in the shoulder may produce discomfort and stiffness, similar to a rotator cuff injury. However, arthritic pain is often more widespread and linked with joint deterioration rather than tendon tears.

• Biceps Tendonitis: Inflammation of the biceps tendon may cause symptoms similar to rotator cuff injuries, although the discomfort is usually limited to the front of the shoulder and may spread down the biceps.

When To Seek Medical Attention?

Knowing when to seek medical assistance for shoulder discomfort might help you avoid more harm and heal faster.

• If shoulder discomfort continues for more than a few days and does not improve with rest and over-the-counter pain medication, seek medical attention.

• Severe discomfort in the shoulder, particularly after an accident, requires rapid evaluation.

• Limited Function: Difficulty with everyday tasks including dressing, lifting, or reaching above requires medical assessment.

• Weakness or instability in the shoulder may suggest a rotator cuff injury and should be evaluated by a specialist.

• If there is visible swelling, bruising, or deformity in the shoulder, see a healthcare practitioner to rule out significant injuries.

Individuals may ensure prompt and successful rotator cuff injury care by detecting symptoms, comprehending diagnostic processes, distinguishing between similar diseases, and knowing when to seek medical assistance.

CHAPTER 3

Non-Surgical Treatment Options

Physical Therapy Exercises

Physical therapy is often the primary line of treatment for rotator cuff issues. It aims to strengthen the shoulder muscles, increase flexibility, and restore function. A physical therapist creates a customized workout regimen based on the patient's ailment and physical condition.

1. Range of Motion Exercises: These exercises are designed to restore normal mobility in the shoulder joint. Simple activities such as pendulum swings, which involve leaning forward and swinging your arm in short circles, may help you retain flexibility. Shoulder stretches, such as the cross-body stretch, which involves pulling one arm across the body and holding it with the other, may also be therapeutic.

2. Strengthening Exercises: Rotator cuff muscular strength is essential for healing and injury prevention. Exercises such as internal and exterior rotations with a resistance band might be beneficial. For external rotations, connect the resistance band to a doorknob, grasp it with one hand, and pull your arm outward. Similarly, for internal rotations, bring your arm inward across your torso.

3. Scapular Stabilization Exercises: Strengthening the muscles around the shoulder blade (scapula) aids shoulder mobility. Commonly advised exercises include scapular squeezes, in which you press your shoulder blades together, and rows, in which you draw a resistance band or weight towards your body while keeping your elbows close to your sides.

4. Maintaining appropriate posture is critical for reducing tension on the rotator cuff. PT sessions often include posture-improving exercises, such as standing or sitting with your shoulders back and down, as well

as chin tucks, which involve pulling your chin gently back to align your neck with your spine.

Regular and continuous involvement in PT exercises may greatly improve shoulder function and minimize discomfort, generally avoiding surgery.

Anti-Inflammatory Medications

Anti-inflammatory medicines are routinely used to treat pain and inflammation caused by rotator cuff injury. These drugs minimize swelling and pain, enabling patients to participate more fully in physical therapy and everyday activities.

1. Nonsteroidal anti-inflammatory drugs (NSAIDs) include ibuprofen (Advil, Motrin) and naproxen (Aleve), which are routinely prescribed or accessible over the counter. They act by blocking the enzymes that cause inflammation and discomfort. It is important to adhere to the dose guidelines advised by

healthcare experts to prevent possible side effects such as gastrointestinal problems or cardiovascular risks.

2. Topical anti-inflammatory creams and gels, such as diclofenac (Voltaren), may be administered directly to the shoulder region. They give regional pain and inflammatory alleviation while avoiding the systemic negative effects of oral drugs.

3. **Acetaminophen:** Although not an anti-inflammatory, acetaminophen (Tylenol) may be used to treat pain. It is often advised for people who are unable to tolerate NSAIDs. To avoid liver damage, do not exceed the prescribed dose.

4. **Prescription drugs:** In extreme instances of pain, physicians may prescribe stronger drugs, such as prescription-strength NSAIDs or pain relievers. Due to the potential for adverse effects and dependence, these drugs should only be administered under strict supervision.

Patients should review their pharmaceutical choices with their doctor to identify the best treatment strategy for their specific requirements and medical history.

Corticosteroid Injections

Corticosteroid injections are an effective way to reduce inflammation and discomfort in the rotator cuff. These injections provide corticosteroids, which are potent anti-inflammatory drugs, directly to the afflicted region.

1. **Procedure:** A healthcare practitioner normally administers the injection, which is frequently done under ultrasound supervision to guarantee precise placement. The region is cleansed, and a local anesthetic may be administered to numb the skin. To decrease inflammation, a corticosteroid is injected into the rotator cuff or adjacent bursa (a fluid-filled sac).

2. Corticosteroid injections may give considerable pain relief, enabling patients to engage more fully in

physical therapy and other non-surgical therapies. The results vary, with some people seeing relief for many weeks or months.

3. Corticosteroid injections are normally administered just a few times per year due to the possibility of adverse effects such as tendons and cartilage weakness. Overuse of these injections may result in problems, thus they are often used as part of a larger treatment strategy.

4. **Considerations:** Corticosteroid injections, although beneficial in lowering inflammation and discomfort, do not treat the rotator cuff injury's underlying etiology. They work best in combination with physical therapy and other therapies that attempt to strengthen and rehabilitate the shoulder.

Patients should explore the advantages and dangers of corticosteroid injections with their doctor to see whether this medication is appropriate for their unique illness.

Lifestyle Changes And Activity Adjustments

Lifestyle and activity changes are critical components in managing rotator cuff problems and preventing future damage. These adjustments lessen shoulder tension and improve recovery.

1. Avoiding Overhead Activities: Activities that require repeated overhead motions, such as painting or carrying heavy things over one's head, may aggravate rotator cuff issues. Patients should reduce or avoid these activities until their shoulder heals.

2. Ergonomic adjustments on the job or at home may help to decrease shoulder tension. Adjusting the height of a computer display to eye level and sitting in a chair with sufficient back support may assist in maintaining normal posture and avoiding shoulder strain.

3. Using Assistive Devices: Devices such as shoulder braces or slings help support and immobilize the shoulder, enabling it to rest and recover. These should be administered under the supervision of a healthcare expert to prevent reliance and muscle atrophy.

4. Weight Management: Keeping a healthy weight helps lower the total pressure on the shoulder and enhances healing results. A healthy diet rich in anti-inflammatory foods including fruits, vegetables, and omega-3 fatty acids may also aid in recuperation.

5. Gradual Return to Activities: When resuming activities, it is critical to go gradually. Patients should begin with low-impact exercises and gradually increase the intensity as shoulder strength and flexibility improve. This method helps to avoid re-injury and improves long-term healing.

6. Regular follow-up with a healthcare professional is required to assess progress and make any changes to the treatment plan. Patients should contact their physician as soon as they notice any new or worsening symptoms.

Patients who incorporate these lifestyle and activity changes may help the healing process and lower the chance of future damage, making non-surgical treatment alternatives more successful.

CHAPTER 4

Preparation For Surgery

Initial Consultations And Evaluations

The first step in preparing for rotator cuff repair surgery is to meet with your orthopedic specialist. This appointment usually includes a complete medical history review and physical examination. The surgeon will inquire about your symptoms, their length, and how they impact your everyday activities. They will also ask about any past shoulder injuries or operations, as well as any other medical problems you may have.

During the physical exam, the surgeon will evaluate your shoulder's range of motion, strength, and stability. To determine the amount and severity of your rotator cuff damage, you may need to undergo specialized tests such as the empty can test or the drop arm test.

Imaging investigations are a critical component of the assessment process. To rule out bone abnormalities or arthritis, your doctor may request X-rays, as well as an MRI, which provides comprehensive pictures of the rotator cuff tendons and muscles. The MRI allows the surgeon to better assess the size, position, and severity of the tear, which is critical for surgical planning.

An ultrasound is sometimes employed as a diagnostic tool, providing a dynamic image of the soft tissues of the shoulder. Based on these examinations, the surgeon will decide if surgery is the best choice and, if not, will offer other therapies.

Instructions And Preparations For Preoperative Care

Once you and your surgeon have decided to continue with surgery, you will be given precise pre-operative instructions.

These suggestions are intended to ensure that the process runs well and to decrease the possibility of difficulties.

Medication Adjustments: Your surgeon may evaluate your current prescriptions and may advise you to discontinue some drugs, such as blood thinners or anti-inflammatory medications, to lower the risk of bleeding during surgery. It is critical to give a comprehensive list of all medicines, including over-the-counter meds and vitamins.

Fasting Requirements: You will most likely be asked not to eat or drink after midnight the night before your procedure. This fasting helps to avoid aspiration (breathing in food or drinks) during anesthesia.

Medical Clearance: Depending on your general health, you may need approval from your primary care physician or a specialist, especially if you have chronic diseases such as diabetes or heart disease.

This might include further testing including blood work, an EKG, or a chest X-ray.

Arranging Transportation and Support: Because you will be unable to drive following surgery, prepare for someone to transport you to and from the hospital or surgical facility. It's also helpful to have someone remain with you for the first 24-48 hours after surgery to assist with everyday routines.

Home Preparations: Create a pleasant healing environment at home. This might involve keeping frequently used goods within reach, planning meals ahead of time, and arranging for help with housework and personal care. Make sure you have ice packs and any recommended medicines ready to use.

Understanding The Risks And Benefits Of Surgery

It's important to understand the possible dangers and advantages of rotator cuff repair surgery. This understanding allows you to make a more balanced choice and prepares you for the healing process.

Benefits

Pain alleviation: One of the key advantages is great pain alleviation. Many patients report reduced shoulder discomfort, which enhances their quality of life.

Improved Function and Strength: A successful surgery may restore shoulder strength and function, enabling you to resume everyday activities, employment, and sports that were previously hindered by the ailment.

Repairing a torn rotator cuff may help avoid subsequent shoulder injury and consequences like arthritis or tendon retraction, which can develop if the rupture is not repaired.

Risks

Infection: Although uncommon, there is a chance of infection at the surgery site. Your surgical team will take steps to reduce this risk, such as employing sterile methods and maybe administering antibiotics.

Nerve Damage: There is a slight chance of nerve damage during the treatment, which might cause numbness, weakness, or discomfort in the shoulder and arm.

Stiffness and Loss of mobility: Post-operative stiffness is frequent, and physical therapy is essential for restoring complete mobility. Patients may have prolonged stiffness despite rehabilitative attempts.

Re-tear: There is a chance of the tendon tearing again, especially if the previous year was big or if the patient resumes intense activity too soon.

Setting Realistic Expectations For Recovery

Understanding the rehabilitation process and having reasonable expectations are critical to a good result. Recovery after rotator cuff repair surgery is slow and may take many months.

Immediate Post-Surgery: Your arm will be in a sling to preserve the repair and restrict mobility. Pain and swelling are usual in the first few days, and your doctor will prescribe pain medicine to alleviate the discomfort.

Physical Therapy: Physical therapy is an essential component of healing. It usually starts with passive exercises, in which a therapist rotates your arm to maintain flexibility without aggravating the repair. As you recuperate, you will graduate to active activities to regain strength and function.

Recovery Timeline: Recovery periods vary, however, most patients should anticipate wearing a sling for 4-6 weeks, starting light activities around 6-8 weeks, and beginning strengthening exercises around 3 months. Full recovery, including resuming all activities, might take 6-12 months.

Compliance and Patience: Following your surgeon's and physical therapist's recommendations is crucial. Avoiding intense activity and following recommended workouts can help you recuperate faster and avoid issues. Patience is essential since speeding the process might result in setbacks or re-injury.

Understanding these processes and thoroughly preparing can allow you to undergo rotator cuff repair surgery with confidence, knowing what to anticipate and how to best ease your recovery.

CHAPTER 5

Surgical Procedures For Rotator Cuff Repair

Arthroscopic Surgery

Arthroscopic surgery is a less invasive treatment for repairing rotator cuff injuries. During this operation, the physician makes tiny incisions around the shoulder, usually three or four. These incisions, which are approximately the size of a buttonhole, allow for the insertion of a small camera known as an arthroscope and specialized surgical equipment.

The arthroscope sends real-time video pictures to a display, providing the surgeon with a good view of the shoulder joint's inside. This improved imagery aids in accurately finding the rip and determining its size and severity. Using the little devices placed via the other incisions, the surgeon may then make the repairs.

The repair method consists of numerous steps:

1. Debridement: The removal of damaged or torn tissue around a rip.

2. Tendon mobilization is gently moving the damaged tendon back to its natural attachment point on the bone.

3. Anchoring involves attaching the tendon to the bone using suture anchors. These anchors are little screw-like devices that are implanted into the bone. Sutures linked to the anchors are then run through the tendon and tightly secured to keep it in place until it heals.

Arthroscopic surgery is preferred owing to its low invasive nature, which often results in less post-operative discomfort, faster recovery periods, and smaller scars than standard open surgeries.

Open Surgery

Open surgery, also known as classic rotator cuff repair, involves making a wider incision across the shoulder to have direct access to the torn rotator cuff muscle. This procedure is often utilized for severe or intricate rips that would be difficult to heal arthroscopically.

An open surgical approach involves the physician making a 6-10 cm long incision to expose the shoulder joint. The deltoid muscle is gradually divided to provide access to the damaged tendon. This open method enables the surgeon to feel and touch the tendon directly, making it simpler to treat major injuries or reconnect the tendon to the bone if it has retracted extensively.

The repair procedure in open surgery is identical to that of arthroscopic surgery.

1. Exposure and Debridement: The surgeon removes any damaged tissue around the tear.

2. Tendon Mobilization: The damaged tendon is moved back to its original attachment location.

3. Anchoring: Sutures are utilized to repair the tendon to the bone, often with the assistance of suture anchors.

While open surgery may be a more easy way to treat complicated rips, it usually results in a longer recovery time, greater post-operative discomfort, and a wider scar.

Mini-Open Repair

Mini-open repair incorporates components of both arthroscopic and open surgical approaches, attempting to balance the advantages of each approach.

This procedure uses a smaller incision than regular open surgery, often about 3-5 cm.

The operation starts with an arthroscopic examination and debridement of the shoulder joint, similar to the completely arthroscopic approach. Following the preliminary arthroscopic procedure, a tiny open incision is made to improve access for the real repair.

The steps involved are:

1. **Arthroscopic Preparation:** The surgeon uses the arthroscope to clear out the injured tissue and evaluate the tear.

2. **Mini-Open Incision:** A minor incision is created to improve access to the damaged tendon.

3. Tendon mobilization and repair include mobilizing the tendon and anchoring it to the bone using sutures and suture anchors.

This procedure combines the direct vision and handling features of open surgery with less invasiveness of arthroscopy, resulting in a moderate recovery time and fewer scars than standard open surgery.

Choosing The Right Surgical Approach

The ideal surgical technique for rotator cuff repair is determined by various criteria, including the extent and complexity of the tear, the patient's general health, activity level, and personal preferences.

• Arthroscopic surgery is ideal for minor to medium-sized tears and individuals who want a quicker recovery time and less scarring. It is also appropriate for people who may be unsuitable for more intrusive treatments owing to other medical issues.

• Open surgery is ideal for severe, complicated injuries or when the tendon has retreated extensively from the bone. It is also explored for individuals who have had prior procedures or have extensive muscular damage.

- **Mini-Open Repair:** Ideal for people who need the advantages of both techniques. It allows for direct tendon manipulation while being less invasive than full open surgery, making it a reasonable option for mild injuries.

Surgeons assess each patient's condition, taking into account criteria such as the size of the tear, tissue quality, patient age, activity level, and personal objectives. A detailed conversation between the patient and the surgeon helps in making an educated selection of the most appropriate surgical method.

CHAPTER 6

Post-Surgical Recovery And Rehabilitation

Immediate Post-Operative Care

Following rotator cuff repair surgery, urgent post-operative care is critical for a full recovery. During this stage, patients are often carefully observed in a recovery room or surgical unit before being released home or to a hospital. The immediate priorities are to control pain, avoid problems like infection or excessive bleeding, and maintain the patient's stability before proceeding with the healing process.

Patients may have pain and discomfort shortly after surgery, which is typical. Pain management techniques, such as surgeon-prescribed medication, cold packs, and elevation of the afflicted arm, are often used to ease these symptoms.

In addition, the surgical site will be bandaged or covered to preserve it and reduce swelling.

During the first healing phase, patients must adhere to any particular recommendations issued by their surgeon about wound care, medication use, and activity limitations. These guidelines may differ based on the kind of surgery done and the patient's specific requirements. Following these rules may assist promote healthy healing and lessen the likelihood of problems.

Physical Therapy And Rehabilitation Exercises

Physical therapy and rehabilitation activities are essential in the healing process after rotator cuff repair surgery. While it is critical to allow the surgical site to heal initially, early mobility and mild movement of the shoulder joint are often recommended to minimize stiffness and enhance circulation.

A physical therapist will collaborate with the patient to create a customized rehabilitation plan based on their unique requirements and objectives. This strategy may include a mix of passive range of motion exercises, active-assisted activities, and strengthening exercises for the muscles that surround the shoulder joint.

Initially, therapy sessions may concentrate on modest motions to assist regain shoulder mobility and flexibility while minimizing stress on the healing tissues. As the patient's condition improves, the intensity and complexity of the exercises may be progressively increased to build shoulder strength and stability.

Consistency and devotion to the rehabilitation program are critical to attaining the best results. Patients are usually urged to do their recommended exercises at home in between treatment sessions to reinforce the gains they achieved during official rehabilitation. With time and effort, most patients may restore full function and range of motion in their shoulder after rotator cuff repair surgery.

Pain Management Strategies

Effective pain management is critical throughout the healing period after rotator cuff repair surgery. While some discomfort is expected following surgery, severe or poorly controlled pain may impede recovery and significantly impair the patient's overall experience.

To successfully treat pain, surgeons may prescribe a mix of medicines, including over-the-counter pain relievers like acetaminophen or nonsteroidal anti-inflammatory drugs (NSAIDs), as well as prescription-strength pain relievers like opioids for more severe cases.

In addition to medicine, various pain management measures may be used to reduce discomfort and improve recovery. These may include the use of ice packs or cold treatment to minimize swelling and numb the surgical site, as well as pain management and relaxation strategies such as deep breathing exercises.

Patients should talk freely with their healthcare providers about their pain levels as well as any concerns or adverse effects from their pain management regimen. Patients and healthcare professionals may collaborate to design a personalized strategy for pain management that promotes comfort while reducing the risk of side effects or consequences.

Monitoring Progress And Preventing Complications

Monitoring progress and recognizing possible issues are critical steps in the post-operative healing process after rotator cuff replacement surgery. Patients should be careful in monitoring their symptoms and notifying their healthcare practitioner of any concerned changes or difficulties that develop throughout their recovery.

Infection, severe bleeding, stiffness, paralysis, and nerve damage are among the most common consequences of rotator cuff repair surgery. By regularly monitoring for signs and symptoms of these issues, healthcare practitioners may react quickly to avoid future difficulties and encourage optimum recovery.

Patients should also schedule any necessary follow-up meetings with their surgeon or primary care physician to check their progress and address any questions or concerns. During these sessions, the surgeon may do physical exams, imaging studies, or other testing to assess the healing process and verify that the shoulder joint functions correctly.

In addition to medical monitoring, patients may take proactive actions to improve their recovery and reduce the chance of problems. This may involve strictly sticking to their recommended rehabilitation program, adhering to activity limits, keeping a healthy lifestyle, and avoiding habits or activities that place excessive strain on the recovering shoulder joint.

Patients who take a proactive approach to monitoring progress and avoiding problems may improve their results and recover successfully after rotator cuff repair surgery.

CHAPTER 7

Complications And Risks Of Rotator Cuff Surgery

Common Surgery Complications

Rotator cuff surgery, like other surgical procedures, has risks and problems. While these problems are uncommon, it is important to be aware of them before undertaking the surgery. Infection is a frequent complication. Despite thorough sterile procedures in the operating room, there is always a possibility of bacterial contamination resulting in infection at the surgical site. Infection symptoms may include pain, edema, redness, warmth, and drainage from the incision site. If you encounter any of these symptoms following surgery, you must immediately tell your surgeon, since early action is critical to avoiding future problems.

Another possible risk is nerve damage. The nerves around the shoulder are sensitive and may be accidentally injured during surgery, resulting in symptoms including numbness, tingling, weakness, or lack of feeling in the arm or hand. Nerve injuries are infrequent, but they may have serious implications if not treated immediately. Your surgeon will make efforts to reduce the chance of nerve damage during the surgery, but you should discuss this possible consequence with them beforehand.

There is also a danger of blood clots developing in the veins of the arm, known as deep vein thrombosis (DVT). This risk is increased in people who have a history of blood clots, obesity, or extended immobility. DVT symptoms might include edema, discomfort, warmth, or redness in the afflicted arm. If left undiagnosed, DVT may lead to significant problems such as pulmonary embolism, so get medical assistance if you notice any unusual symptoms following surgery.

Other possible side effects of rotator cuff surgery include shoulder stiffness, weakness, or chronic discomfort. These difficulties might be caused by scar tissue development, insufficient healing, or underlying shoulder arthritis. Physical therapy and rehabilitation are critical components of the post-operative healing process because they assist reduce problems and restore strength and range of motion to the shoulder.

Recognizing Signs Of Infection Or Re-Injury

Following rotator cuff surgery, it is critical to examine the surgical site for symptoms of infection or re-injury. Infection may develop despite careful sterile precautions in the operating room, so it's critical to be aware of any signs that may signal a problem. Infection symptoms may include increasing pain, edema, redness, warmth, or discharge from the incision site.

If you encounter any of these symptoms, please tell your surgeon right once so that proper therapy may be begun.

In addition to infection, there is a danger of rotator cuff re-injury after surgery. This may happen if the repaired tendon is exposed to too much stress or pressure before it has had time to recover properly. It is critical to closely follow your surgeon's post-operative instructions to prevent actions that might damage the repair's integrity. This may involve wearing a sling to support the shoulder, avoiding heavy lifting or overhead tasks, and undergoing physical therapy to progressively rebuild the shoulder muscles.

If you suffer a rapid onset of significant pain, weakness, or instability in your shoulder after surgery, get medical assistance immediately, as these might be indicators of re-injury. Your surgeon may prescribe imaging tests, such as an MRI or ultrasound, to assess the integrity of the repair and identify the best course of action.

Dealing With Post-Surgical Stiffness

Stiffness is a typical problem after rotator cuff surgery, and it may have a substantial influence on your ability to conduct everyday tasks and engage in rehabilitation exercises. Scar tissue growth surrounding the repaired tendon is a common cause of post-surgical stiffness, which may impair the shoulder joint range of motion. To treat this condition, your surgeon may prescribe modest stretching and range-of-motion exercises to gradually restore shoulder mobility.

Physical therapy is an important part of the post-operative rehabilitation process because it helps break down scar tissue and improves flexibility and strength in the shoulder muscles. Your physical therapist will collaborate with you to create a rehabilitation program tailored to your requirements and objectives.

Exercise improvement may be gradual at first, but with persistent effort, it will increase with time.

In certain situations, your surgeon may propose further procedures to address chronic stiffness, such as manual therapy methods, corticosteroid injections, or, in rare cases, revision surgery to remove scar tissue or correct the initial repair. However, these procedures are normally reserved for situations in which conservative methods have failed to improve range of motion.

Long-Term Outcome And Prognosis

The long-term results of rotator cuff surgery might vary depending on several variables, including the size and severity of the tear, the quality of the repair, and the patient's compliance with post-operative rehabilitation procedures. In general, most patients have considerable improvements in pain and function after surgery, with the bulk of healing happening within the first six to twelve months.

However, it is critical to set realistic expectations for the healing process and recognize that complete recovery may take time. Some patients may endure lingering shoulder weakness or stiffness even after the first healing phase, especially if the rupture was substantial or there were pre-existing degenerative abnormalities in the shoulder joint.

Regular follow-up meetings with your surgeon are essential for monitoring your progress and addressing any issues or difficulties that may emerge. Your surgeon may prescribe frequent imaging tests, such as an MRI or ultrasound, to assess the integrity of the repair and verify that the tendon is healing appropriately.

Overall, with proper treatment and rehabilitation, the prognosis for rotator cuff surgery is typically excellent, and most patients can resume regular activities with less discomfort and better shoulder function.

However, you must continue to care for your shoulder and follow your surgeon's long-term maintenance instructions to reduce the chance of re-injury and enhance the repair's lifespan.

CHAPTER 8

Enhanced Recovery And Healing

Nutritional Support For Healing

Proper diet is essential for the rehabilitation and healing process after rotator cuff surgery. Your body needs certain nutrients to repair tissues, decrease inflammation, and promote general recovery. A well-balanced diet high in vitamins, minerals, protein, and healthy fats may considerably help in recuperation.

Protein is an essential ingredient for healing. Protein is a structural component of tissues and muscles, hence it is required for rotator cuff healing. Incorporating lean protein sources like chicken, fish, tofu, beans, and lentils into your diet may aid in tissue regeneration and muscle rehabilitation.

In addition to protein, eating meals high in vitamins and minerals is critical for healing. Vitamin C, for example, aids in collagen formation, which is essential for tendon regeneration. Citrus fruits, strawberries, bell peppers, and broccoli are great sources of vitamin C. Similarly, zinc-rich foods such as nuts, seeds, and whole grains may boost the immune system and assist in tissue healing.

Fish, flaxseeds, and walnuts contain omega-3 fatty acids, which have anti-inflammatory qualities and may help decrease inflammation and improve healing. Consuming these healthy fats might help you recover faster.

Hydration is also essential for healing. Drinking enough water flushes toxins from the body and keeps tissues hydrated, which is critical for good recovery. Aim to drink at least eight glasses of water every day, and restrict your intake of sugary and caffeinated drinks, which might impede the healing process.

Role Of Supplements And Medications

In certain situations, your healthcare physician may offer vitamins or drugs to aid in the healing process after rotator cuff repair surgery. These supplements may assist address nutritional gaps in your diet while also providing extra support for tissue regeneration and reducing inflammation.

Collagen is a regularly suggested supplement. Collagen supplements may assist promote tendon and ligament health, which aids in rotator cuff rehabilitation. Supplements containing glucosamine and chondroitin may also benefit joint health by lowering pain and inflammation.

Omega-3 fatty acid supplements, such as fish oil capsules, may provide further anti-inflammatory benefits. However, you should contact your healthcare physician before beginning any new supplement regimen to confirm that it is safe and suitable for your specific requirements.

In addition to vitamins, your doctor may prescribe drugs to help control pain and inflammation throughout the healing process. Nonsteroidal anti-inflammatory medicines (NSAIDs), such as ibuprofen or naproxen, may be used to relieve discomfort and swelling. When taking any medicine, you must carefully follow your doctor's instructions and report any adverse effects as soon as possible.

Importance Of Sleep And Rest

Adequate sleep and rest are required for the body to recuperate adequately after rotator cuff repair surgery. The body goes through many processes during sleep that support tissue repair, muscular development, and general recuperation.

It is critical to emphasize sound sleep by providing a comfortable sleep environment and implementing appropriate sleep hygiene behaviors. Aim for 7-9 hours of unbroken sleep every night to help the healing process. Avoid coffee and electronic gadgets before bedtime since they may disrupt sleep quality.

In addition to sleep, rest times throughout the day are critical for the body's recovery from the stressors of surgery and physical therapy. Listen to your body's cues and take pauses as required to avoid overexertion and encourage recovery.

Psychological Aspects Of Recovery

The psychological side of rehabilitation is sometimes underestimated, yet it plays an important part in the whole healing process. Dealing with pain, limited mobility, and the emotional stress of surgery may all hurt mental health.

It is critical to recognize and treat any emotions of worry, despair, or frustration that may occur throughout the healing period. Seeking assistance from friends, family, or a mental health professional may help you manage these feelings and have a positive attitude toward your recovery.

Relaxation practices such as deep breathing, meditation, or yoga may also aid in stress reduction and emotional well-being throughout the healing process. Stay in touch with your healthcare team and share any issues or problems you may be facing so that they can give the appropriate assistance and advice. Remember that rehabilitation is a lengthy process, so be patient and gentle with yourself to ensure a good conclusion.

CHAPTER 9

Return To Daily Activities And Sports

Gradual Return To Work And Daily Activities

Returning to work and regular activities after rotator cuff repair surgery needs patience, care, and following your doctor's instructions. Your recovery time may differ based on the severity of your injury and the kind of surgery done. In general, you'll begin with passive motions and proceed to active movements as your shoulder recovers.

During the early phases of rehabilitation, it is critical to emphasize rest and avoid activities that may strain your shoulder. Your doctor may advise you to wear a sling to help support your shoulder and minimize mobility. As your discomfort subsides and your range of motion improves, you may gradually resume light activities of daily living, such as dressing and doing modest home chores.

As you heal, you'll progressively increase the intensity and length of your workouts. Your physical therapist will walk you through a personalized rehabilitation program aimed at strengthening your shoulder muscles and increasing your range of motion. It's important to listen to your body and avoid pushing yourself too hard since this might cause setbacks in your recovery.

Returning to work should be done carefully, with an emphasis on gradually increasing your workload and avoiding activities that may strain your shoulder. To facilitate your rehabilitation, your doctor may propose changes to your work environment or tasks. Communicate with your employer about any limits or restrictions you may have, and fight for your health and well-being.

Overall, returning to work and everyday activities after rotator cuff repair surgery needs patience, perseverance, and a willingness to follow your doctor's instructions. By gradually increasing your activity levels and listening to your body, you can ensure a smooth and effective recovery.

Guidelines For Resumed Sports And Physical Activities

To minimize re-injury, it is necessary to prepare ahead of time and follow certain rules while returning to sports and physical activities after rotator cuff repair surgery. Your doctor will make suggestions based on your specific condition, but there are some broad guidelines to follow.

First and foremost, you must wait until your shoulder has completely recovered before resuming sports or hobbies that require repeated overhead movements or heavy lifting. Rushing back too soon may raise your chance of re-injury and extend your healing period.

Once your doctor has approved you to continue sports and physical activities, you should gradually increase the intensity and length of your exercises. Begin with low-impact activities that do not place too much strain on your shoulder, such as walking or swimming, and progress to more difficult exercises as your strength and endurance improve.

Pay careful attention to your body's signals and discontinue any activities that produce pain or discomfort. It is natural to feel stiff and painful when you return to sports and physical activities, but intense or chronic discomfort may signal a condition that needs to be addressed.

It is also important to warm up correctly before participating in any physical activity and to cool down afterward to avoid muscular stiffness and pain. Incorporating stretching and strengthening exercises into your regimen will assist improve flexibility and stability in your shoulder joint, lowering your chance of recurring injury.

Finally, be patient with yourself and allow your body to adapt to the demands of sports and physical activities. It's normal to have setbacks along the road, but with patience and effort, you can gradually recover your strength and confidence on the field or in the gym.

Strategies To Prevent Re-Injury

Preventing re-injury following rotator cuff repair surgery requires patience, good technique, and continuing shoulder care. While it is hard to prevent the danger of re-injury, you may use a variety of measures to reduce your odds of problems.

First and foremost, follow your doctor's rehabilitation advice and gradually resume your usual activities. Rushing back too soon or overexerting yourself may raise your chances of re-injury and lengthen your healing period.

Maintaining proper posture and body mechanics is also important for avoiding re-injury. Avoid slouching or hunching your shoulders, particularly while doing overhead movements or heavy lifting. Instead, keep your shoulders relaxed and your spine straight to alleviate tension on your shoulder joint.

Strengthening the muscles around your shoulder joint is another important part of avoiding re-injury. Your physical therapist may recommend specific exercises to strengthen your rotator cuff muscles and enhance shoulder stability and function. To enhance the efficiency of these exercises, they must be performed regularly and appropriately.

In addition to strength workouts, including flexibility and mobility drills in your regimen may help avoid stiffness and enhance the range of motion in your shoulder joint. Yoga and Pilates, in particular, may help to improve flexibility and body awareness.

Finally, listen to your body and prioritize rest and recuperation as required. Pushing through discomfort or disregarding warning signals of overexertion might result in further injuries and delays in your rehabilitation. It is critical to establish a balance between pushing yourself and allowing your body the time it needs to recuperate and adjust.

By using these measures and keeping diligent in your rehabilitation efforts, you may reduce your risk of re-injury and resume a full and active lifestyle after rotator cuff surgery.

Maintaining Shoulder Health In The Long Run

To maintain shoulder health over time, you must commit to continual care and pay attention to your body's demands. Even after your shoulder has completely recovered from rotator cuff repair surgery, you must maintain excellent behavior to avoid future problems and enhance general health.

Regular exercise is essential for keeping your shoulders healthy and minimizing muscular imbalances and weaknesses that may contribute to injury. Incorporate a variety of exercises throughout your workout to target various muscle groups and improve overall strength and stability in your shoulders and upper body.

It's also critical to monitor your posture and body mechanics throughout regular tasks and exercise. Avoid slouching or rounding your shoulders, particularly while sitting or standing for a long time. Instead, keep your shoulders back and down while maintaining a neutral spine posture to avoid tension on the shoulder joints.

In addition to exercise and posture, an adequate diet is important for preserving shoulder health. Eating a well-balanced diet rich in lean protein, fruits, vegetables, and whole grains may aid in muscle healing and repair while also lowering inflammatory levels.

Regular stretching and mobility exercises may help increase the flexibility and range of motion in your shoulder joint, lowering your risk of stiffness and injury. Before exercising, include dynamic stretches and foam rolling into your warm-up regimen, followed by static stretches in your cool-down routine.

Finally, listen to your body and allow yourself to rest and heal as required. Overtraining or pushing through discomfort may result in overuse injuries and delays in your development. It is critical to establish a balance between pushing yourself and giving your body the time it needs to repair and adapt.

Following these instructions and prioritizing shoulder health in your everyday life can allow you to live a full and active lifestyle for many years to come.

CHAPTER 10

Long-Term Maintenance And Prevention

Regular Exercise Routines For Shoulder Strength

Regular exercise regimens are essential for the long-term maintenance and prevention of rotator cuff problems. They maintain the shoulder muscles strong and healthy. These exercises not only serve to avoid injuries but also improve the general stability and functioning of the shoulder joint.

Shoulder external rotation is a fundamental exercise for developing shoulder strength. This workout focuses on the rotator cuff muscles, namely the infraspinatus and teres minor. You may execute this workout using resistance bands or lightweight dumbbells. Begin by standing with your elbow bent at 90 degrees and your forearm parallel to the ground. Slowly twist your forearm away from your body, maintaining your elbow near your side. Repeat this action for a certain number of times, progressively increasing the resistance as your strength grows.

Another useful exercise is shoulder internal rotation. This exercise targets the subscapularis muscle, which is also found in the rotator cuff. This exercise, like external rotation, may be performed with resistance bands or dumbbells. Begin by standing with your elbow bent at 90 degrees and your forearm parallel to the ground. Slowly twist your forearm towards your body, maintaining your elbow near your side. Repeat this action for a certain number of repetitions, progressively increasing the resistance as required.

In addition to rotator cuff exercises, including general shoulder strengthening exercises in your program might be advantageous. These might include shoulder presses, lateral lifts, and front rises. To prevent stressing the shoulder joint, start with small weights and gradually increase the intensity.

When it comes to shoulder strengthening exercises, consistency is essential. Aim to do these exercises at least two to three times a week, with enough time in between to rest and recover. It's also important to listen to your body and adjust the workouts as required to prevent aggravating any current ailments or pain.

By including regular shoulder strength exercises in your long-term maintenance plan, you may help avoid future rotator cuff issues and maintain ideal shoulder health.

Techniques To Maintain Flexibility

Maintaining flexibility in the shoulder joint is critical for avoiding stiffness and injury. Stretching exercises may increase flexibility and range of motion, allowing your shoulders to remain fluid and useful.

The doorway stretch is a helpful method for maintaining shoulder flexibility.

This stretch focuses on the muscles in the chest and shoulders, which may get tight due to poor posture or repeated motions. To execute the doorway stretch, stand in a doorway with your arms bent at a 90-degree angle and your forearms against the doorframe. Lean gently forward until you feel a stretch at the front of your shoulders and chest. Hold this posture for 30 seconds to one minute, taking deep breaths and relaxing into the stretch. Repeat multiple repetitions throughout the day to reduce tension and increase flexibility.

Another effective method is the shoulder rotation stretch. This stretch stimulates both the internal and external rotator cuff muscles, which helps to increase mobility and reduces the risk of impingement. To do the shoulder rotation stretch, stand with your feet shoulder-width apart and your arms at your sides. Slowly rotate your shoulders forward in a circular motion, maintaining control and fluidity. After a few repetitions, reverse the rotation to target other muscle groups. To keep the shoulder joint flexible, execute this stretch regularly.

In addition to static stretches, dynamic stretching activities may help improve shoulder flexibility. These exercises include rotating the shoulder joint through its whole range of motion in a controlled way, which helps to warm up and prepare the muscles for action. Dynamic shoulder stretches include arm circles, shoulder rolls, and arm swings. Add these stretches to your warm-up regimen before exercise or physical activity to help avoid stiffness and improve shoulder mobility.

Consistency is essential for maintaining shoulder flexibility. Include stretching exercises in your regular regimen, concentrating on static and dynamic stretches to target various muscle groups. Regularly exercising these exercises can help keep your shoulders flexible, mobile, and injury-free.

Tips For Preventing Future Injuries

To avoid future rotator cuff problems, take a proactive approach to shoulder care and maintenance. Certain tactics and lifestyle adjustments may help you avoid the likelihood of reoccurring shoulder issues and maintain good shoulder health.

Maintaining appropriate posture and body mechanics is a key strategy for preventing future injuries. Poor posture may put additional pressure on the shoulder joint, increasing the likelihood of overuse problems and impingement. Be aware of your posture throughout the day, whether you're sitting at a desk, standing, or doing physical exercise. Keep your shoulders relaxed and your spine aligned to prevent stress on the shoulder muscles and joints.

Another important recommendation is to avoid overworking the shoulder joint with repeated or excessive motions. This includes things like hard lifting, overhead tossing, and repeated reaching actions. If you participate in these sorts of activities regularly, be sure to vary your motions and take frequent rests to enable your shoulders to rest and heal. Strength training activities aimed at the muscles around the shoulder joint may also assist improve stability and lower the chance of injury.

It's also critical to listen to your body and recognize any warning signals of impending damage. If you have recurrent shoulder discomfort, weakness, or a restricted range of motion, get medical assistance right once. Ignoring these signs might result in future injury and consequences. A healthcare practitioner can provide an accurate diagnosis and propose treatment choices to address the root cause of the condition.

In addition to these proactive steps, leading a healthy lifestyle may help with general shoulder health and injury prevention. This includes eating a healthy diet, keeping hydrated, getting enough sleep, and controlling stress. By caring for your body and emphasizing self-care, you may improve the health and function of your shoulders while also lowering your risk of future injury.

Regular Check-Ups And Monitoring

Rotator cuff injuries need regular check-ups and monitoring to ensure long-term maintenance and prevention. By being proactive and observant about your shoulder health, you may spot possible concerns early on and take necessary action to remedy them before they worsen.

Schedule frequent check-ups with a healthcare expert, such as a physical therapist or an orthopedic specialist, to review your shoulders' condition and look for any changes or anomalies. During these visits, your doctor may undertake a physical examination, diagnostic testing, and a review of your medical history to assess your shoulder health and identify any risk factors for injury.

In addition to frequent check-ups, self-monitoring is an essential part of shoulder care. Keep an eye out for any changes in your shoulder function, such as soreness, weakness, or reduced range of motion, and seek medical assistance if any of these symptoms persist. Keep note of your activities, including those that aggravate or ease your symptoms, since this information might help you discover possible triggers or risk factors for injury.

Incorporate frequent monitoring into your daily routine by doing self-assessments of shoulder function and range of motion. This might include easy exercises or motions to test your shoulder strength and flexibility, such as reaching high, lifting things, or twisting your arms. If you observe any major changes or irregularities, contact a healthcare expert for additional assessment and advice.

By being proactive about your shoulder health and emphasizing frequent check-ups and monitoring, you may discover and manage any possible concerns early on, ensuring excellent shoulder function and mobility for years to come.

Conclusion

Finally, both medical professionals and patients benefit from a thorough grasp of rotator cuff repair. This complex treatment, which aims to restore function and relieve discomfort in the shoulder, requires a multimodal strategy that includes preoperative evaluation, surgical technique, and postoperative rehabilitation.

First, the preoperative period lays the groundwork for a favorable result. Accurate diagnosis by clinical examination, imaging investigations, and sometimes arthroscopy is critical in identifying the degree of the damage and arranging the right surgical solution. Understanding the patient's medical history, activity level, and expectations is critical for designing the treatment plan to meet their specific requirements.

Surgical technique is critical in rotator cuff repair, with technological developments and surgical methods constantly improving results. Whether doing arthroscopic or open treatments, the surgeon must carefully handle the torn tendon, providing correct tension, secure fixation, and enough coverage. The choice of repair approaches, such as single-row, double-row, or transosseous-equivalent, is determined by many criteria, including rip size, tissue quality, and surgeon preferences. In addition, adjunct treatments such as subacromial decompression or biceps tenodesis may be used to improve results.

Postoperative rehabilitation is essential for successful rotator cuff repair, with an emphasis on regaining range of motion, strength, and function while preserving the healing tendon. A planned rehabilitation regimen, adapted to the particular patient and surgical procedure, directs the progressive transition from passive range of motion activities to active strengthening exercises. Compliance with the rehabilitation regimen is critical to avoiding problems including stiffness, muscular weakness, and re-tears.

Despite advances in surgical procedures and rehabilitation programs, successful rotator cuff restoration is not assured. Patient characteristics such as age, tear size, tissue quality, and rehabilitation compliance all have a substantial impact on results. Complications such as stiffness, adhesive capsulitis, infection, or re-tears may also develop, demanding careful monitoring and therapy.

To summarize, a full grasp of rotator cuff repair includes all aspects of treatment, from preoperative examination to surgical intervention and postoperative rehabilitation. Clinicians may enhance outcomes and quality of life for people with rotator cuff disease by combining evidence-based therapy with tailored patient care. As the profession evolves, continuous study and innovation will help us better understand and treat this prevalent shoulder issue.

THE END